HEALTHSCARE

HealthScare
CONFESSIONS OF A
HOSPITAL SPIN DOCTOR

CLAY DeSTEFANO

Laurence –
Enjoy the read!

Clay
DeStef

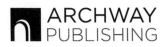
ARCHWAY
PUBLISHING

Archway Publishing books may be ordered through booksellers or by contacting:

Archway Publishing
1663 Liberty Drive
Bloomington, IN 47403
www.archwaypublishing.com
1 (888) 242-5904

Because of the dynamic nature of the Internet, any web addresses or links contained in this book may have changed since publication and may no longer be valid. The views expressed in this work are solely those of the author and do not necessarily reflect the views of the publisher, and the publisher hereby disclaims any responsibility for them.

Any people depicted in stock imagery provided by Thinkstock are models, and such images are being used for illustrative purposes only.
Certain stock imagery © Thinkstock.

ISBN: 978-1-4808-1940-5 (sc)
ISBN: 978-1-4808-2461-4 (e)

Library of Congress Control Number: 2015918946

Print information available on the last page.

Archway Publishing rev. date: 11/18/2015

Dedication:

To Anne, Mom and Dad—may your personal stories, and those of others I have shared here, help to inspire all who read them accordingly.

June 29, 2016

Hi Uncle Lawrence,

I finally got you a copy of the health book I mentioned. (And it's signed by the author! :-)

Also, a belated thank you for the memorial gift in Dads honor.
We made a donation to the Central Texas Life Care (crisis pregnacy center). They do a great job counseling young women to keep their baby and not have an abortion. They do good work and appreciated the contribution!

Hope you're having a good summer.

Dan

126-2

I finally got you a copy of the (health) book I mentioned, (and it's signed by the author!)

Dana

CONTENTS

PART 1:

THE OTHER SIDE
OF THE FENCE

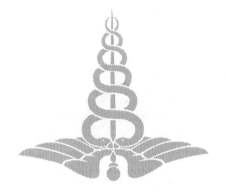

CHAPTER 1
THE GREAT AND POWERFUL OZ

My wife, like my father and many other Americans, is a health care *junkie*. She believes in doctors, pills, shots, implements—even surgical intervention—for *everything*. It's been a running debate between us for our entire thirty-plus-year marriage.

Two winters ago she began experiencing strange pain in her stomach, followed by vomiting and diarrhea. The flu-like symptoms continued off and on for a few weeks.

By spring, they were back and worse. This time whenever she changed position—from lying flat to sitting up, standing from sitting, or going up or down stairs—she'd be hit with excruciating pain, followed by vomiting and diarrhea.

Despite my hesitation, she insisted that I go out of town to attend a corporate training seminar. While I was away, her condition worsened, and a friend took her to the emergency room of the hospital where I worked. She was treated for pain, given fluids, and run through some additional tests. Her case was a bit of a mystery because she was displaying a variety of symptoms but no definitive diagnosis could be given. She was discharged and referred to a gastroenterologist for follow-up.

When she couldn't get in to see any of the specialists on our medical staff quickly enough, she and her friend decided to go to the hospital in the next town. By the time I returned from my trip, my wife was scheduled for a study to check out her gallbladder function. She underwent the test, and it showed that her gallbladder wasn't functioning properly.

After reviewing the test results, the gastroenterologist informed me that her gallbladder needed to come out and he could fit her into his surgical schedule the next day in Austin. My wife immediately said she wanted it taken out. I explained to the doctor that I was employed by a different hospital and asked if he could perform the procedure there. He told me he didn't practice there, didn't know anyone who did, and he promptly hung up on me.

Apparently once he realized he wasn't going to make any more money off of us, he was done. No referral, no hand off, just a click on the other end of the phone.

I called one of the surgeons on our medical staff that I admired and trusted and asked if he would be willing to give us a second opinion. He graciously agreed to see us that same afternoon. He asked several questions and reviewed her records and the same study the gastroenterologist had. He told us that even though her gallbladder function wasn't normal, she didn't have any of the other classic symptoms to suggest it needed to come out.

Amazingly enough, *this* surgeon was not recommending surgery.

When I explained that the condition had been going on for nearly thirty days nonstop and my wife had lost almost thirty pounds in that time, he made a phone call to one of the gastroenterologists on our medical staff, who also graciously agreed to see us that same day. While this gastroenterologist also could find no immediate medical reason for the symptoms, it was clear that her health was precarious, so he admitted her for "failure to thrive."

A few hours later, she was in a bed in our hospital scheduled for more intensive testing. In addition, she was on IV fluids, pain control, and a liquid diet. The immediacy of the attention certainly made her feel better emotionally, and the IV and pain meds temporarily masked her physical symptoms.

After a few days, the best diagnosis seemed to be vasculitis NOS (not otherwise specified). She was discharged and referred to a rheumatologist for further testing and treatment.

We were told that vasculitis was an inflammatory disease that comes in different forms. In her case it seemed to be inflaming the veins and arteries that fed her digestive system.

The rheumatologist's treatment consisted of a combination of steroids and other anti-inflammatory drugs. The steroids worked remarkably well; however, due to numerous side effects, it was not recommended that she stay on them for an extended period of time. For a while she responded to the cycled up, down, and eventually off steroid treatment.

Then we moved on to the big guns—a chemotherapy drug that has had good results with long-term anti-inflammatory treatment.

Despite my hesitancy, my wife was game.

To me, it was hard to tell which was making her sicker—her condition or the stated side effects of the drugs she was on. I wanted her to get off the drugs, but she had read and been told that the treatment could take three or more months before you would see any improvement.

She persevered.

Soon we were on to a pain-medicine specialist, who initially prescribed immediate-release morphine. When those were no longer effective, he transitioned her to extended-release morphine and was about to write a prescription for a wheelchair because she was too weak and doped up to walk.

That's when I objected the loudest.

Winter was nearly upon us again, and in less than a year's time, my wife had gone from seemingly healthy to almost having unnecessary gallbladder surgery; regularly ingesting a chemotherapy drug, along with round-the-clock morphine; and now she was about to succumb to a wheelchair. All of this so-called progress occurred while she was under the care of medical specialists.

By then we'd already spent thousands of dollars and invested nearly a year of our lives in finding a fix, and from my perspective, things were worse than when we'd started.

My wife and I were emotionally and physically exhausted and desperate to find a better solution. I asked for a referral to one of the leading diagnostic and treatment centers in the country. The rheumatologist was now serving as my wife's primary care provider and agreed it was a good idea. He helped arrange the appointment, and within a few weeks, we were on our way.

We arrived late in the day on a Wednesday in early December— just in time to do a little reconnaissance on the campus so we'd know where to be for our first set of appointments that began at seven thirty the next morning.

Despite the inhospitable weather, we could not have felt more welcome or safe. We picked up a wheelchair in our hotel lobby. The chair would stay with us the entire trip and be my wife's salvation. It would be mine as well. The chair made it possible for her to be mobile without triggering an attack.

As snow fell and the Christmas lights of the mega–medical complex twinkled from across the street, we settled into our room for the night.

The facility's campus—in fact the whole community—was warm and friendly. From the physicians and support staff to the shop clerks, waitresses, and even locals on the street, all seemed incredibly oriented toward the patients of the facility and the loved ones accompanying them.

A series of pedestrian skyways and subways connect the buildings of the medical complex with hotels, restaurants, and shopping malls so you never have to go outside if you choose not to.

The assorted buildings that make up the medical facility's campus itself are filled with world-class artwork. You hear concert-quality music coming from a grand piano in the main lobby. And despite its vastness and the thousands of people walking through the common halls and accessing care along with you, the beautiful architecture, healing light, and meditative spaces help to calm and reassure you that *you're in the right place* for whatever it is that ails you.

Everyone seems to be focused only on *you.*

The facility's customer service rivals the best of any four-star hotel. People are warm, kind, patient, and incredibly helpful. I was both amazed and delighted to discover such a culture existed in modern health care, because I'd always been told by my superiors that I expected too much of our customer-relations efforts. They'd claim that health care environments were too complex; there were too many people and touch points to be able to consistently deliver compassionate, quality service *each* and *every* time.

This place not only excels at it, their culture permeates the *entire* community. Even the cab drivers and airport personnel are friendly and focused on you!

Over the next several days, my wife saw a number of specialty physicians, underwent a battery of tests, and even had a minor skin cancer removed. Their ability to juggle multiple physicians, testing, and procedures on an as-needed basis is remarkable. Her appointments changed several times while we were there in order to accommodate her needs, and we never waited more than thirty minutes for anything.

I was so impressed with their efficiency and attentiveness that I didn't object to having them run duplicative lab and imaging tests and repeat procedures from the past few months, even the detour to the dermatologist for the skin cancer, I felt OK about all of it because, after all, this was the Great and Powerful Oz.

We had not made arrangements to stay beyond a week, so we returned home to Texas without a definitive diagnosis. A referral to have a particular imaging test performed that was considered the gold standard for diagnosing vasculitis was the key to solving the mystery.

Exhausted, grateful, and hopeful, we returned home and celebrated a happier Christmas than originally anticipated. We gladly spent New Year's Eve having the final imaging test performed that promised to provide our final answer to what had been plaguing her for nearly a year. Results were to be sent to her specialty team at the facility, and we would then determine the best and most appropriate treatment. All the while my wife remained convinced that her situation would improve only through the hands of these clinicians.

The initial feedback from the interventionist on the day he performed the test in Austin confirmed what we already knew. A couple of the main arteries that fed my wife's stomach had some blockage; however, it was seemingly not enough to cause her symptoms.

We held on to the hope that our new, expensive, out-of-town specialists would see something different, and we waited to hear more.

A few weeks passed, and we hadn't heard from them. My wife placed a phone call and sent an e-mail through the online patient portal to her primary care physician there. After a few more days, we finally heard that the test had been lost in transmission and they had asked for it to be sent again.

Several more weeks passed, and still no answer came.

In the meantime, we had received our bill for our portion of the visit, which was not covered by insurance. It was nearly $4,000. This was followed by two separate appeals for donations to the facility's foundation.

Still no results came, and I opted to hold off on paying our share of the bill until they did.

A new statement arrived each month in the mail, but no updates or responses to our inquiries did. I finally called to say I had no intention of paying the bill until one of our treating physicians called us with some sort of report. Even though I knew in my heart that they had nothing new to tell us, it was a matter of principle for me now. I was told that my wife's primary care physician had "tried to call her several times but was not able to reach her."

Really? My wife had been in bed or on the couch with her phone by her side for the past seventeen months. I couldn't imagine how she could have missed a call. Even if she had, I wondered why they didn't use voicemail. When we were on site, they called both of our phones regularly and left voicemails if we didn't pick up.

By then it seemed painfully obvious that even the leading health care facility in the country is only focused on you when you are present and paying for the appointments, tests, and procedures they so effectively and efficiently arrange in your presence.

The next statement we received showed that it took four months for the imaging study performed in Texas to arrive and be read by the facility's specialist, and we had been charged an additional $717 for this *deplorable* service.

At this point I felt that because there was no more immediate money to be made off of my wife's care; their white-glove service had deteriorated to the same dysfunctional series of miscommunications, ball-dropping, and finger-pointing, as it does for almost every other health provider in America today. I had mistaken their culture of providing excellence in care services with *caring*.

We heard from her doctor shortly after my call—only to be told what we *already knew*. Since several month's had now passed since the study, at the doctor's suggestion, my wife underwent another imaging test at our local hospital to compare the artery blockages and see if the vasculitis had progressed.

Thankfully, it had not.

To me, the entire experience ended up being nothing more than a very expensive, frustrating, and inconclusive second opinion. I remain more convinced than ever that the current model for receiving health care in America is horribly broken. It's ineffective. It's bankrupting too many with little or no return. And worst of all, it's designed to keep Americans dependent on it.

Winter was upon us yet again. Nearly two years had passed since my wife's vasculitis symptoms began. She'd now lost more than seventy pounds since the onset of the symptoms.

She remained committed to traditional medical treatment.

The condition continued to debilitate her on a daily basis. She was completely off steroid treatments but even more heavily into the chemotherapy drug, which I was now begrudgingly injecting into her belly "fat" once a week.

I felt more hopeless and helpless than ever.

As another New Year arrived, my wife was too weak to resist, and as I was now her 24–7 caregiver, I started her on an extremely restrictive anti-inflammatory diet in addition to the variety of vitamins and supplements she's been regularly taking to combat the effects of the dangerous and powerful drugs.

We had a two-month follow-up visit with her rheumatologist three weeks later. According to his analysis, her overall health status had worsened since her last visit. (Again, we paid someone to tell us what we already knew.) I insisted that the chemotherapy drug was making her sick and she needed to get off of it. To my relief, her doctor agreed. They settled on a less-dangerous prescription treatment in her latest round of Rx Roulette, and we made a follow-up appointment to see him again in two months. That same day we also received our latest invoice from Oz, followed by a separate appeal in the mail a day later to donate to their foundation.

Ten months have now passed. My wife remains largely on an extremely healthy anti-inflammatory diet, which has produced some amazing results. She has stopped taking *all* of her prescriptions. Essential oils are a part of her regular routine, and she's becoming more physically active each day. She researched, found, and purchased CBD (raw hemp) oil online. It has also made a significant difference in her health. She's actually done some light cooking and cleaning for the first time in two years. Her symptoms have lessened in intensity and frequency and continue to do so. She's beginning to leave the house more and more. We've taken a few short trips, and she's even gained a few pounds.

I feel great and sick at the same time.

I'm more convinced than ever that the modern American health care system is the primary culprit in the current, horrible state of health most Americans are living in today. I feel terrible and disgusted to know that over the past three decades, I have helped to create, sell, and promote modern health care as something that it *isn't*.

I can't remain quiet. *Mea culpa.* I owe it to my soul and the American public to confess my sins and omissions.

Chapter 2
Eyes Wide Shut

"**A**re you a doctor?"

"No," I would generally reply with a smile each of the hundreds of times I was asked.

"You look like one," was the normal follow-up, almost always then followed by a very personal, health-related question posed to me—the nondoctor—about the person's care.

Because of the way I look and talk, people are willing to have me provide care for them—no questions asked.

Crazy but true.

There is little doubt in my mind that most people's need to have *someone else* fix their health issue(s) for them is the underlying problem causing such poor health in America today. Like all of their other personal responsibilities, too many individuals are willing to turn their health over to anyone in a lab coat or someone who even *looks like* a health care provider.

While I spent nearly three decades as a "spin doctor" for hospitals and doctors, I seldom used either personally. In fact, I do my best *not* to. I avoid the modern medical industrial complex and lately, its coconspirator, the food industrial complex, in all its forms.

Medical intervention can be necessary and helpful; however, I've also seen, heard, and experienced enough to know that it also cannot.

I believe medical care should be sought only as a last resort and even then, with extreme caution. More specifically, when accessing and purchasing health care, buyer beware.

Unfortunately, Americans today seem addicted to health care and all its spin-off industries, and like our other addictions, it's killing us.

I've always believed in and personally practiced a healthy, preventive lifestyle. Regrettably, most Americans do not want to be accountable for their own health. They do not seem willing to take responsibility for their choices any more than they are willing to own up to other consequences of their actions.

Worse, too many people today engage in the modern health care system with their eyes wide shut.

Never was this clearer to me then when I rounded on patients in their hospital beds or talked with friends and loved ones about their various health concerns. I am constantly amazed at how little most people know about and participate in their own heath. From bad lifestyle choices and horrible eating habits to not taking simple preventive measures, *most of us are responsible for our current state of health.*

While it's tempting to blame doctors, hospitals, big pharma, insurance companies, and politicians for all our country's health woes, the truth is Americans themselves are as culpable as the rest.

The problem with placing the responsibility of improving and maintaining your good health *solely* in the hands of a doctor is there are good doctors and bad ones, and without a little effort on your part, it's hard to tell the difference.

It's also important to note that the modern health care system is focused on *caring for the sick.* Keeping you well is *your* responsibility.

By and large, doctors—just like insurance companies, big pharma, and hospitals—make decisions based on the economic impact to their business.

Will I/we make money?

Will I/we lose money?

The truth is doctors practicing medicine today are living in a time that has never been more personally demanding or rapidly changing. Practically everything they know and do in their daily practice of medicine is in *constant* motion.

They make money from seeing patients who don't require a lot of their time or effort. (Sick patients are generally less productive for them.) Continuing insurance reform is making it harder to make good money only by seeing and treating patients. That's why so many doctors today are also owners of ancillary businesses like freestanding clinical labs, imaging centers, and/ or surgery centers. Others still receive additional income serving as medical directors for freestanding facilities, from outpatient treatment services to nursing homes and beyond.

I'm sure you are thinking, "This is America. Shouldn't doctors be allowed to be entrepreneurial and make money too?"

In theory, yes, but when the fox is guarding the hen house, we all know what happens to the hens. Unfortunately, more often than you may realize, when a doctor today tells you that he/she wants new labs or X-rays to review, very often it's because he/she stands to *profit* from your use of these services too.

They will often use the line, "I don't trust that facility" or "Those records are a few months old. I'd like you to have it done again here." Most patients comply (including my wife and me during her visit to the world renowned medical facility) because most believe their doctors wouldn't order tests if they weren't *necessary*.

Last year my ninety-one-year-old mother needed to change her primary care physician and cardiologist because her previous ones were both retiring. Her new physician was affiliated with a different hospital and immediately ordered a battery of tests, including an imaging study. Mom was not your typical ninety-one-year-old, compliant patient. She explained to the new doctor that she had undergone most of these tests in the past few months and didn't want to put herself through the stress and expense of these additional and, in her mind, unnecessary tests. The doctor agreed on the labs but pushed back on the imaging study.

When she responded, "I'm ninety-one. Regardless of what you find, I have no intention of putting myself through any additional procedures or surgery, so why bother?" the doctor couldn't argue.

She also skipped finding a new cardiologist, because I explained that her minimal heart issues could be monitored just as effectively by her new primary care physician, which would save her time, money, and duplicate testing.

She didn't have the tests and recently went back for a six-month checkup. Her new doctor said her numbers were better than ever. In fact, now that she is no longer seeing a separate cardiologist, they're considering taking her off some of her meds ...

In February we helped Mom celebrate a healthy ninety-two. We just returned from a quick visit where she again inspired all of us with her beauty, vitality, and mental faculties. Don't get me wrong, I definitely saw an elderly woman who has physically aged and slowed down dramatically since our last visit, but as Mom repeatedly states whenever our conversations inevitably turn to health, "Come on, after all, I'll be ninety-three in February, which means I'll actually be starting my ninety-*fourth* year. I'm old."

On the flipside, my father grew up in a family of pharmacists. At one point they even owned a private, retail pharmacy. Like my wife and many other people, Dad was a health care *junkie*. He was convinced that there was a pill, spray, salve, brace, device, shot, or medical intervention for whatever ails you.

While he was alive, he wanted every test, procedure, and "miracle cure" his doctors had to offer. Despite the fact that he was in his mid-eighties, already legally blind from macular degeneration, and in rapidly declining health due to a massive stroke he had suffered six years earlier, his eye specialist helped convinced him (granted, it didn't take much) to undergo special injections in his eyes monthly. The injections, which held the promise of potentially improving his macular degeneration, were expensive and not covered by Dad's insurance. With each injection Dad's blood pressure soared, his bank balance declined, and his vision did not improve.

The same doctor next helped convince Dad that he was potentially a good candidate for a new surgical trial he was conducting. Once again, Dad happily signed on. I insisted on joining him and Mom on his next visit with his primary care physician. When I told Dad's doctor that he was planning to undergo eye surgery, his doctor alarmingly explained that, due to his poor health, Dad would more than likely die on the table. He did not have the procedure and lived a few more years without any major incidents.

Is it wrong for doctors to push care and procedures from which they may financially benefit?

While there are differing opinions on this, my answer is yes, *if* the test/procedure is not medically called for. So who makes *that* call? Well, regrettably, most often it's that pesky fox (doctor) again.

Imagine trying to run a profitable business that is based on providing care to a certain number of patients using protocols and systems that are constantly changing and very often designed by others who don't practice in the field. Huge debt—little to no control; not the game you thought it was and constantly changing rules, regulations, and reimbursement rates ...

Does any of this sound like a *winning recipe* for a happy, successful work environment?

That's why so many doctors today are frustrated and seeking to be employed by large medical groups and hospitals. They want financial security. They want *someone else* to take the risks. They want *normal* lives.

Of those who do not want to be employed or give up control, many are abandoning their traditional specialty, such as obstetrics and genecology, for just gynecology—and turning to cosmetic reconstructive gynecology at that.

Others still are dropping out of standard insurance/payment models altogether to treat a set number of patients of their choosing for a flat monthly fee.

Lots of doctors are offering procedures and products that aren't necessarily included in their board-certified specialty.

They are expanding their retail offerings and exploring new ways to provide care and services *not* covered by insurance directly to consumers willing to pay *out-of-pocket* to look younger, thinner, whatever.

America was built on the free-enterprise system, but health care wasn't. Any successful business owner learns to give the public what it wants; however, health care isn't a commodity to be developed and changed by the whims of the fickle American public.

Without proper controls and restraints, more providers will likely move away from the mundane, repetitive, and un/less-profitable services to only the bright, shiny, profitable ones.

This mentality is already contributing to an alarming and growing shortage of primary care doctors/providers in America. Doctors and other providers have to be focused on our health and well-being because, largely, *we aren't*. In addition, when doctors are spread too thin and only focus on making money, *bad* things often happen.

Americans were shocked to learn of Joan Rivers' premature death in the fall of 2014. But as more of the facts unfolded, her story was no different than that of thousands of our friends, loved ones, and neighbors.

A freestanding, outpatient facility without proper controls; a doctor focused on money rather than his patient's health; a consumer focused on convenience over character, competence, and credentials ... a tragic end that is repeated throughout America every day.

We only heard about the Joan Rivers tragedy because of her celebrity.

As business owners, savvy doctors are going to give you what you want. They will perform procedures when they are not medically called for. They will prescribe medication and write orders for tests and therapies because you want them. Like any successful service provider, doctors who want to make money will do everything in their power to keep you happy, satisfied, and returning for more.

Thankfully, there are exceptions, but truthfully the consumer-driven growth in health care services is changing the face of health care and *not* in a good way.

America's addiction to fix/change me now health care is only fueling the fire.

Consumers also need to open their eyes to the fact that doctors and other health care providers are just as distracted, unhappy, and disinterested in their jobs as many other Americans seem to be. Really, how focused on *you* do you think these men and women are?

Think about it. How often do you have great paid encounters with anyone in a service industry—a salesperson, waitress, mechanic, store clerk? The work ethic in America today seems to have eroded to a level of "I could *not* care less about you or this job, and I'm only going through the motions because it's the best I can muster up right now."

Now think about the doctors, nurses, technicians, and other support staff involved in your care process. They too are human just like you and me. They are working for a paycheck when they are *caring for you*.

Your wellbeing—maybe even your life—depends on understanding this. Do *not* confuse the business of providing care to you with caring *about* you!

In fairness, there are *many* caring, engaged doctors, nurses, and techs in the field; however, the standard working conditions most perform within are not conducive to sustained compassionate, engaged care.

Doctors work challenging hours. Many are on call 24-7 Most are sleep deprived or compromised.

In the hospital setting, most nurses work twelve-hour shifts. That means they can potentially work "a full week" in three days and do it again somewhere else another two or three days a week. For many, this temptation to make "good money" is too hard to resist. The added stress on their bodies, emotions, personal and professional relationships and you—their patients—may not currently be under study; however, I'm convinced it is also a bad model for all.

Caregiver-to-patient ratios are based on the nurses' employers' economics, *not* outcomes. Mandatory behaviors and increasingly popular scripted rounds all add up to a challenge for even the most caring among them.

Now think about the nonclinical support staff that assists providers with carrying out the tasks of overseeing and delivering your care. That same disinterested, distracted attitude that results in your fast food order *not* including the fries you ordered leads to miscommunication, mistreatment, and countless bad outcomes in doctors' offices and health care facilities throughout America every day.

In 2006 the hospital industry kicked off a national patient safety initiative called One Hundred Thousand Lives. The goal was to stop and reverse the alarming trend of preventable medical errors that was killing one hundred thousand Americans each year. In 2014, a new study published in the *Journal of Patient Safety* stated that revised numbers are now over four hundred thousand unnecessary deaths in hospitals each year, making medical errors the *third leading cause of death* in the United States. And that number only reflects hospital deaths. The figure doesn't reflect unnecessary deaths in doctors' offices, freestanding clinics, etc., because there is less regulatory oversight in these settings, so tracking of this does not occur with any consistency.

Where's the outrage?

Where's the Senate investigation?

Where's the bucket challenge?

New government-required models utilizing electronic medical records and menu-driven, best practices have yet to demonstrate their value to improving the overall health and well-being of Americans. At the same time, undeniable evidence is piling up left and right that our current health care model is broken and in desperate need of *true* reform.

Truthfully, bad medical outcomes are not entirely the doctors' and other providers' fault. American health care consumers are largely asleep at the switch.

Equally disengaged consumers/patients are major contributors to their own demise. In fact, more than 80 percent of the diseases and illnesses Americans are being treated for today, including out-of-control diabetes and heart disease, are mostly self-imposed through poor lifestyle choices.

This recipe for disaster is compounded by the fact that America is aging at a faster rate than ever before and obesity—along with all of the health-related complications and comorbidities it brings—is already at epidemic levels.

We can and must do better.

Health care consumers have to become better informed and actively participate in their own health. Doctors need to learn to respect and empower their patients for healthy, two-way relationships. And growth and free enterprise in health care needs to be monitored and properly supported. If we are going to truly change delivery systems and improve patient outcomes, we have to change the way by which we purchase, access, and pay for health care.

Because current payment (insurance) models only pay for traditional, recognized therapies and procedures, true innovation, free enterprise, and further exploration into alternative treatments needs to be fostered, incentivized, and ultimately paid for by insurance companies.

PART 2:

THE BUSINESS OF HEALTH CARE

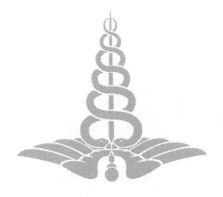

CHAPTER 3
BIG STUFF

Like most children who grew up in the '60s and '70s, my perception of doctors and health care in general was primarily shaped by limited personal encounters, television shows, and Norman Rockwell illustrations. On TV *Ben Casey, Dr. Kildair,* and *Marcus Welby* were all depicted as highly engaged, compassionate advocates for their patients. Warm and loving images of kindly old general practitioners and their happy patients graced the walls of doctors' offices, calendars, and many magazines of my childhood.

This subtle messaging helped to shape the perception that doctors are good guys who are devoted to you, their patient. Impression after impression made you believe that *your* health is paramount to *your* physician, and everything else in his world takes a backseat.

It wasn't until the late '70s that we began to see doctors portrayed as the complicated and multidimensional *human beings* they really are. With that, however, drama trumps reality on TV and in film, so these complicated bad boys and girls you came to admire on shows like *St. Elsewhere, ER,* and *Grey's Anatomy* were and are still depicted as much more superhuman and compassionate than most in my experience.

I entered into the health care field in 1984 when I joined the community relations department of a hospital owned by the leading for-profit hospital company in America. This particular facility was among the corporation's flagships at the time and featured the atypical model of a closed medical staff. The hospital's medical staff was made up almost entirely of a single, multidisciplinary group practice of nearly one hundred primary and specialty care physicians who owned and operated the group that was physically attached to the hospital. One of my primary functions was to serve as the community relations liaison between the hospital and this subspecialty medical group.

I was twenty-five years old, my wife and I were expecting our first child, and I had found an opportunity to do "meaningful, important work." I honestly believed it was a privilege to serve among these *super-humans*.

My reeducation began on my first day as I encountered a physician on an elevator during a tour with my new boss. The physician introduced himself using his first and last name, so naturally I said. "It's very nice to meet you, Jack." He smiled and shook my hand, and with that the elevator door opened and he stepped off.

I don't think the doors had fully closed before my boss shouted, "*Never* call a doctor by his first name!"

So ended my first lesson.

This rule was only the first of many idiosyncrasies of the physician culture I was to learn. I'm going to spare you the details; however, here's the cliff-noted version: in health care doctors *rule*. They are treated as a special class that is not required to play by the same set of rules the rest of us do.

Granted, most businesses and industries are fraught with elite/special interest groups. The difference is in health care the protection, lack of accountability, and rewarding of bad behaviors is costing people their well-being and in some cases, their lives.

Our corporation was making big strides in the business of health care, and our facility was no exception. One of our surgeons was in training for the Jarvik 7 ® artificial heart program, and I was given the plum job of writing a feature piece about it in the corporate journal.

Barney Clark and Bill Schroeder were household names thanks to their Jarvik 7® artificial heart procedures. Things were still looking promising for the device, and our surgeon had been training in the program for nearly two years. He had successfully implanted the device into several calves, and when we sat down for the interview, the forty-three-year-old Yale graduate had bragging rights for the longest survival rate among training program calves with implanted devices.

Because of our success with the artificial heart training program, I accompanied the *CBS Morning News* crew that came to our ER one night to follow a potential heart attack patient through initial diagnosis and treatment. Not long afterward we began clinical trials for the then-pioneering hearing device the cochlear implant.

Big stuff. I was less than a year into this gig, and I was writing for a national publication and working with the *CBS Morning News*!

In the same year, the baby my wife and I were expecting became the cover model for our new childbirth advertising campaign; we opened two new hospitals and celebrated the tenth anniversary of our main facility.

Fast times.

Fun times.

And admittedly, a bit too bright and shiny for me to see what was really going on.

Chapter 4
Into the Fire

Halfway through my second year with the for-profit giant, the physician group with which we were affiliated decided to create its own health maintenance organization. Managed care was beginning to change reimbursements to doctors, and these guys wanted to control the impact of it.

The group was pleased with my work as their community relations liaison and wooed me away from the hospital to become their *first-ever* director of communications.

The year was 1986. The group was a multispecialty practice of nearly one hundred physicians that fancied itself as a Mayo-like facility. To date, my exposure to physicians had been limited and I thought, *What's not to like?*

Ultimately, my immaturity and ego overruled my gut, and I accepted the position. I soon found out that working occasionally *with* doctors was very different from working *for* them.

My first project was to improve on our communications (i.e., signage, telephone directories and other collateral materials used by our patients). We started with a telephone directory. Naturally, I created it in alphabetical order by medical specialty first and then last name, first name, alpha-sort under that. You know, B follows A and so on ... just like we all learned in early grade school.

The proposed patient telephone directory was submitted during my official introduction to the entire physician group at one of its regular shareholders meetings. (The way this particular group was set up, each of the physicians in the group was an equal voting partner. They became voting partners after being voted in by their peers following a twelve-month trial period as nonvoting associates.) All decisions that involved spending any money were approved by a vote of all partners.

What an introduction.

I honestly thought I was going to be fired on the spot. They were red-faced, with voices raised, and totally indignant over the fact I would have the audacity to promote doctors in any way. (Another one of the idiosyncrasies of physician culture at the time was "Doctors *don't* promote themselves."). My offense was made all the worse by the fact that I created the telephone listing in alphabetical order versus their preferred method of *seniority*.

You read right. In the world of doctors, it's all about seniority. Much like academia, deference is paid to the oldest, longest-tenured physicians so, naturally, they expected the telephone directory to mirror the chronological order that the various physicians and then individual specialties incorporated into the group.

Never mind the fact that we had physicians on our staff treating everything from allergies and arthritis to urology. They wanted to start the patient directory with gynecology because one of the founding members of the group was still practicing, and he was a gynecologist/obstetrician. After much debate, I remained employed, but the directory was shelved.

I felt like Dr. Spock—trying to understand the logic of these foreign beings I was among. I soon learned and continued to learn over and over that common sense and logic seem to have no place in the world of doctors.

Proposed updates to the main floor directory I was also working on at the time were halted for the same reason. As unbelievable as this was to me at the time, it paled by comparison to the things I heard and saw over the couple of years I worked for this group.

I understood that as a privately owned practice this group had the right to create and live by its own policies and protocols;

however, the ones this group chose to enforce said a great deal to me about who they were and how they viewed the world.

Unfortunately, there seemed to be nothing noble, humble, or helpful about any of it. In fact, I believe this type of elitism—which still exists today—contributes to the reality that physicians are *not* to be respected or followed *simply* because of their MD.

The truth is doctors are little more than body mechanics, and just like auto mechanics, they are not all created equal. An MD, a white coat, and a stethoscope do not necessarily a competent doctor make.

I've never met a doctor who did not feel that he/she was the best in his/her field. Confidence and bravado is what helps propel many to become doctors. It's also what can make them so dangerous, once they do.

In health care, just like every other world, power, control, and money all have the power to ultimately corrupt.

CHAPTER 5
THE BOYS CLUB

The shareholders' meetings featured four-star gourmet dinners served on starched-white table linens. Only the finest wines, imported nuts, cheeses, and caviar, along with the best cuts of meat, poultry, and offerings from the sea, were served. While the group enjoyed their fine meal and wine, they would make business decisions, including who was approved as a partner and who was not.

Just like in Grisham's *The Firm*, if an associate didn't fit in (i.e., think/act like all the others), he ultimately would not be approved as a partner.

Although I'm not aware of them having anyone taken out, their actions and words were just as *brutal*. This was a boys' club. They played hardball all day, and being in the deep South, it was a good ol' boys' club.

And speaking of boys and *The Firm*, boys will be boys, so there was also an older guy on staff whose primary function was to make sure new recruits were shown a good time during their visit(s) to the facility.

I remember watching in horror and amazement as some of the best and brightest of the new recruits washed out because of their new ideas, methodologies, and in some cases, greater success over a senior partner, and that simply could not be tolerated.

CHAPTER 6
IT'S A DIRTY BUSINESS

Doctors are first and foremost business owners. Most make decisions based on the economic impact on their wallets. In the world of doctors, patients can be and are "fired." Hospitals do it as well. Many a shareholders' dinner included a discussion about no longer serving a certain patient.

Payment issues, difficultly to please, being high-risk for bad medical outcomes, etc., are the reasons most often cited when considering the firing of a patient, and the requests are very often approved.

In the mid-1980s, the quest to make *more* money, or at least prevent potential losses, led the group for which I worked to create their own HMO. They felt they'd have more control over their income because they had enough primary and specialty care providers to cover most medical issues, which would allow them to keep the cost of providing care down. They also had a good financial arrangement with the hospital to which they were attached, so they could control their exposure to loss even more.

Suffice it to say, the story behind the development, widely successful implementation, and ultimate sale of the HMO is a book in itself, but the most important takeaways for me were:

- Don't believe everything an insurance company's or health plan's advertising promises.

- *All* insurance companies rewrite policy on a regular basis—based on their experiences (losses).

Everything in the insurance world is about making money—even more so than on the care side of the business. Insurance companies make no bones about it. That's why they continue to report record earnings year after year while ratcheting down the scope of coverage they provide and ratcheting up premiums and copays for their customers.

The entire process of utilizing your health benefits is designed to make it difficult for you to utilize your coverage. Preauthorizations, explanation of benefits, additional paperwork you receive asking to clarify whether your claim is related to an auto accident—all of these hurdles are ways insurers create challenges and barriers for you to easily access the coverage for which you are paying.

I've seen and heard enough throughout my career to convince me that insurance companies will stop at nothing to keep from paying a claim, but perhaps the most striking was when one of the new HMO's members who was under our care went into premature delivery and ended up in a high-risk obstetrics unit in a competitor hospital.

Her new baby was in the same facility's neonatal intensive care unit. The doctors had not anticipated such an eventuality when creating their HMO, so they had no special financial arrangements with that particular hospital, so they had to pay *full freight.*

The same day the young mother and her baby were hospitalized, the doctors insisted that a new policy be written stating in essence that if a pregnant mother was not enrolled for family coverage by her fifth month, her unborn baby would not be covered for anything at the time of its birth—including the cost of the birth and any related expenses.

They were not going to make this mistake again.

Ultimately, the group decided they did not want to be in the insurance business and sold their successful operation to a commercial insurer.

CHAPTER 7
THE THIN WHITE LINE

first learned about the thin white line then, too.

Doctors, like any fraternity, protect one another. Throughout my career, I have encountered many physicians—even been asked to showcase some in promotions—who had a number of well-documented, questionable outcomes.

While covering for one another to protect mutual interests in not unique to health care, the potential and very real harm these actions cause is much more significant. The very idea that most humans are capable of self-policing is lunacy. Sure, there are some honorable and disciplined among us who walk the straight and the narrow. But daily scandals in the national headlines show us many do not.

Business, politics, law enforcement, professional athletics, finance, higher education, organized religion—pick a group and you'll find countless examples of how we as humans continue to fail to do the right thing.

Personal and collective denial happens in each of our daily lives. It's one of the ways we cope. Millions of compromised elderly drivers get behind the wheel of a four thousand–pound killing machine each day while their loved ones, friends, and sometimes physicians turn a blind eye. Recognizing your own faults, or that your cognitive skills and physical abilities aren't what they once were, requires a kind of honest introspection most of us are incapable of.

The very notion that doctors are different ... better ... more honorable than everyone else is just simply untrue. Doctors protect one another because it's in their best interest to do so.

Hospitals protect doctors because, depending on the specialty, doctors help hospitals make money. Conversely, they can also blacklist a hospital and encourage their colleagues to do the same. Doctors are the lifeblood of hospitals, and the really smart ones use it to their full advantage.

At best, doctors and hospitals are most often *frenemies* who, despite their differences, will work together to protect one another from a liability like you.

So there it is—another ugly truth of the business of health care. Doctors and other health care workers protect one another. Hospitals protect doctors and their other staff. And not many are *truly* looking out for *you*.

CHAPTER 8
I'M OUTTA HERE

The intimate view my job afforded me into the world of doctors allowed me to learn my most important lesson. Doctors are *people*. They are not superhuman. Doctors are not gods. They are not all-knowing. They are not all good guys. They are not all good at their craft. Like all of us, they make mistakes. Many make bad choices. Others make careless, misinformed and/or limited decisions about *your* health.

They are surviving each day just like you and me. And like us, many struggle with relationship problems. They are not immune to life's challenges. Often their teenage children are just as impossible and hateful toward them as yours are to you. Many are living beyond their means. Others are just as technologically challenged by their iPhones, tablets, and the rest of the digital world as you are.

The truth is, once I saw behind the curtain, I immediately lost my *automatic* respect for doctors. I worked then and have since worked with some very good doctors who were also very good people. But in my experience, they were and have been the exception.

The majority of the doctors in the group ultimately moved past their initial objections to being promoted. Before long we had developed a logo and a radio jingle and were regularly advertising on radio and in various local and regional print publications. The efforts paid off handsomely. The group grew from 99 to 120 physicians, and we also added several new medical specialties, services, and locations and a successful HMO to their business holdings.

Despite my success and the group's progress, the more we grew and prospered, the more conflicted I felt about it. Back then, on any given day I might have a doctor or two who was very pleased with me, which meant that more than one hundred others—along with their nurses, wives, and girlfriends—were not. This hero one minute, bum the next, "I love you. I hate you" existence got old.

Eventually, the temper tantrums, extortion tactics, affairs, selfishness, contempt for one another, and ultimately, *greed* got to me.

Watching these guys pontificate from the floor was like having a ringside seat in the US Congress. Seeing their day-to-day actions and maneuverings to improve their personal situations seemingly at the expense of everyone else—including their own partners—was amazing.

I learned so much about people, politics, and power. It was truly the best education I've ever had. It was also the hardest thing I've ever done professionally.

After a year and a half of this daily crazy, anything could have triggered my departure, and of all things it was a dream that did. Here it is just as clearly as I recalled it when I awoke the next morning more than twenty-five years ago …

> I awake to the sound of splashing water. It's coming from the bathroom. I know the kids are too young to reach the sink, so I get up to investigate.

> I creep to the door and open it just enough to see a miniature version of my boss sitting on the edge of the sink. He is naked. His back is turned to me. He is bathing.

> As if seeing an eighteen-inch version of a naked, balding, obese, sixty-something man isn't scary

enough, I'm shocked to notice that he has a tail with a barb at the end. He turns just in time to see me and my shock.

He knows I saw his tail! And now that he's facing me, I can see the two horns on his head!

With that the mini-devil-boss squeals, jumps to the floor, and darts toward the kids' bedroom—grunting, squealing, and feverishly whipping his tail along the way. I somehow manage to grab his tail and throw him down the stairs.

After a few quick laps around the dining room table, he makes a dash toward the stairs—toward the kids! I again somehow manage to grab the barb at the end of his tail, swing him around over my head a few times, fling open the front door, and whip him out into the street ...

Don't judge. I'm sure dream interpreters and psychologists alike will have a field day with that one. The thing is, I don't often recall my dreams, and this one was so vivid and specific that I *simply couldn't ignore it.*

I turned in my resignation the next day and vowed never to seek employment in the health care industry again.

PART 3:

IN THE NAME OF THE FATHER

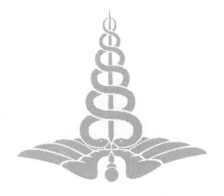

CHAPTER 9
HOLY WORK

Almost ten years passed before I returned to health care employment. I enjoyed a good run with a couple of public relations/advertising agencies and did a stint as an in-house marketing department for one of my former agency clients. Because of my experience, I was given the health care clients at the agencies, so I maintained a connection to what was happening in the industry.

The recession in the early '90s was particularly hard on ad agencies, so you can imagine my delight at spotting a notice for a writing position in the public relations department of a little Catholic hospital in town.

Perfect.

I was raised a Catholic. I knew the drill. I would be working at the hospital—not for doctors—which I enjoyed the first time around. It was a nine-to-five job, so I'd be spending more time with my family, which had grown to five plus two dogs. But most appealing to me, it was a not-for-profit, faith-based hospital.

I was certain that this would make it *different* from my experience with the doctors. I mean, there were sisters in habits walking the floors.

Initially everything I thought the job would be was true. The culture was very different from the doctor group. And by and large, the hospital staff and many of the medical staff worked *there* because of it.

The fact that we had real live daughters of charity walking the halls inspired many of us to focus on service. Like me, many of my colleagues, the care staff and especially our volunteers were drawn to the mission aspect—*doing good works*—of the facility and because of it, there was a kinder, gentler spirit in the air. We were attracted to the purposeful work and the servant-leader culture the sisters fostered to keep it so.

I was grateful to the daughters for connecting me to this compassionate and very real aspect of my former faith. I was especially pleased to meet this particular model of nun as, other than my first-grade Sunday school teacher, a beautiful young novice who sang and played the guitar, every nun I had known prior to this seemed to be the stereotypical angry and mean old lady.

The job was perfect for me. I wrote press releases, newsletters, and ad copy for the facility and its services. I became an expert on the nearly hundred-year history of the hospital.

I used every opportunity to work the story of the daughters, the mission—*the good work*—into internal and external messaging, and it worked. It motivated staff. It comforted patients. And it made the sisters *very* happy.

My arrival at the little Catholic hospital on the hill coincided with the arrival of the hospital's first lay CEO. Prior to his arrival, all the CEOs at this particular hospital had been daughters of charity. And we'd had some real stars. A couple went on to be major players in the national health care arena.

My near-simultaneous arrival with this new CEO also coincided with the opening of a new women's and children's hospital. The unique design, collaborative partnerships with outside entities, and subsequent promotional efforts that followed began an unparalleled period of growth and progress for this health ministry.

Mergers and acquisitions soon changed our owners from the daughters to a new, more corporate entity. Fewer sisters, more accountants, and unbridled growth ultimately transformed the facility into a regional giant and one of the darlings of the newly formed corporation.

When I first arrived, we had eight sisters living on campus. That soon dwindled to five then three and then, eventually, the last sister, a relatively young one whose energy, youth, and expertise could be put to better use elsewhere in the daughters' world, pulled up stakes and officially turned over the reins to the *all-lay staff.*

Despite plenty of notice and a few years of intensive mission integration training, in which I played a direct role, the immediate cultural shift that occurred with the departure of the last sister was so abrupt that most of us could have filed a workers' comp whiplash claim.

I soon found myself squarely back in the boys' club.

Through it all, I learned a great deal. I reconnected with the concept of a higher power. I honed my nonprofit and public service skills. I learned that hospital CEOs are little kings in their worlds, and most should *not* be given the keys to the kingdom.

I also learned that nuns are *people* too.

I was disappointed to learn that most doctors were still jerks and still ruled the health care universe.

And last, I learned that even in the faith-based health care world, power and money *trump* God.

CHAPTER 10
GOD'S SOLDIERS

The daughters did an amazing job of focusing and furthering their culture. If faith-based service to others is what drove one to work at their ministries, all the training, imagery, and language certainly helped to keep one there.

We received extensive orientation as well as ongoing training and leadership development monthly for nearly the entire ten years I worked there.

Each year all two hundred–plus leaders in the organization would gather in the chapel to participate in a recommitment ceremony in order to reconnect with our purpose. We always knew the sisters wouldn't be around forever, so many were happy with and comforted by these rituals. In preparation for their eventual departure, we also worked hard to create a permanent virtual presence of the daughters.

As we grew, the facility offered new venues to showcase our history and culture. Tributes to the sisters were created throughout the main campus and repeated at off-site facilities, including stained-glass art, heritage displays, heroic-sized bronze sculptures, and an abstract sculpture at the main entrance that would have the sisters keeping vigil over us *forever*.

I was honored to play a significant hand in all of it. My contributions to preserving and furthering our culture of caring were recognized and rewarded throughout my tenure.

In addition to serving the sisters directly, I also served on the multifacility task force that helped develop and implement a new set of core values and corporate mission statement for all of the ministries under the new corporation.

I became a trainer and regular presenter of our servant leadership training programs. I also codeveloped and taught an award-winning guest relations program based on the same.

I was so engaged in telling the story of our *good work*, why it mattered, and how each of us could do more to further it that I *truly* didn't notice that we weren't *all* there for the same reasons.

In fairness, the primary focus of my job was to advance and protect the reputation of the facility. I *had* to believe the stuff I was writing, saying, and selling or I couldn't have done it each day.

I chose to work on committees and projects that were mission-focused, and as much as possible, I surrounded myself with likeminded peers. By and large it worked.

We weathered many storms as a leadership group and company, and with each one I felt we became stronger and tighter. September 11 was *huge* in furthering our team spirit and culture. The tragic events that day kicked off a series of town talks, memorials—including singing choirs and videos—and the ultimate "Red, White and Blue Days" that went on for many Fridays following the attacks.

We also learned how to deal with life-threatening crisis of our own *right at home*. The hurricane seasons of the mid-2000s were particularly hard on the Gulf Coast. Three major storms hit our community and facility directly in less than twelve months during the 2004 and 2005 seasons. I was amazed by and proud of my two hundred–plus leader colleagues as we all pulled together to make it work for our staff, our patients, our greater community, and eventually, one another.

Many, including my family, were without power, water, and phones at one point or another. The first storm to hit—Ivan—was a category 3. He struck in the darkness of night, took out twenty-thousand homes, destroyed many businesses, devastated the downtown area, and eliminated access to essential clean water and power for most of the region.

In our case it was twenty-one days before we had power or television at home, yet we all rose above our own challenges for the *greater good,* and most seemed honored to do so.

We were *required* to work before, during, and after the storms. Our focus was to maintain all systems and/or bring up all those that failed as quickly as possible. As the public information officer, I not only participated in but also sat in and reported on everything that happened. The work was fast-paced, unpredictable, and edgy. It was also fun and invigorating.

The outcome was this feeling of amazing connection—a bond with those who worked shoulder-to-shoulder with you—that felt unbreakable.

From my perspective it was easy to feel like you were part of something good and something *very* important.

CHAPTER 11
SISTER ACT

There was little doubt that for most of us, the sisters were an integral part of who we were and what we did each day. They were so beloved that tributes to them by staff were many. One in particular—a small volunteer choir group made up of staff and at least one actual daughter—took it to a new level. The ragtag, a cappella choir donned mini-habits and performed at various hospital-related celebrations and functions a la Whoopi Goldberg and the girls.

For me, the culture of the daughters and my devotion to it was made all the stronger because of the nature of my job. My daily functions included writing promotional materials and producing videos, speeches, letters, and press releases all to advance and protect their wonderful work.

About halfway through my tenure, I was asked by our VP of faith and mission, a younger and more progressive sister, if I would be willing to serve the daughters' community directly in their ancestral home. Of course I said yes and traveled to and fro over a period of a year to assist their community.

We were tasked with developing a logo and strategic plan to help ensure that their works stayed *true* and their many ministries— from health care to education to international humanitarian aid— would continue with or without the sisters' direct involvement.

The sad reality was that the wonderful ministries of the daughters were being forced to turn management responsibilities over to lay people because there simply weren't enough American Daughters of Charity left to run all of them.

There weren't even enough daughters in the workforce any longer to cover the VP of mission and faith post at all of their hospitals, let alone keep them in the CEO slots.

It was very important that we crafted a message and collateral materials that would contribute to the seamless integration of their culture of servant leadership and mission service to each of us, the lay leaders and staff now tasked with running their ministries.

What an honor.

I had no idea what to expect when I arrived late on a snowy New Year's Day at the Emmitsburg campus of the Daughters of Charity. I began my orientation with a tour of the museum dedicated to their founder, Saint Elizabeth Ann Seton. The tour included a quick, private peek at the original home/school/hospital these remarkable early American women created.

The buildings of the facility served as a museum, event center, dormitory, church, and home to retired and infirm daughters. With the exception of the original historic structures, the facility had the feeling of all the Catholic buildings of my youth: lots of stone, stained glass, carved wood, and images of the suffering Christ.

Technically, it was still the Christmas holiday, but decorations were sparse and conservative. Aside from an expansive nativity collection that peppered the windowsills throughout the long halls connecting the dining hall, guest quarters, and common areas, it didn't feel like Christmas at all. It also didn't feel anything like our hospital ministry back home.

My guest quarters, like the rest of the facility, were clean and complete but dated and Spartan. By comparison, the lavish executive suite at our hospital, along with our meeting facilities, IT/AV capabilities, and catering services, were on par with a fine hotel. At the hospital, everything was new, and only the best would do.

My education into the world of the daughters began with our first meeting when I was introduced to my fellow committee members via an interactive strategic session I facilitated to clarify our mission, goals, and objectives.

I quickly learned that these ladies were humans just like you and me. Crazy I know, but my earlier Catholic teaching tended to make one believe that nuns and priests are better, holier people.

Noble.

Catty.

Selfless.

Petty.

Funny.

Not.

Humble.

Proud.

Engaged.

Exhausted.

Young.

Old.

Brave.

Frightened.

I heard and saw it all in that room and during our subsequent team ups over the next year. I came to admire and respect these women all the more for it. I was relieved to learn that they were *human* because that meant their devotion to their faith and work was a choice they made every day.

I enjoyed all the more the "romantic" Valentine's dinner I shared with a few of the sisters at an Italian restaurant in

Baltimore's little Italy, during which they "disparaged" fellow dinners, our servers, and may God forgive them, Frank Sinatra.

During our farewell dinner, I empathized with their disappointment in their community's leaders who bowed to the only comment made by the priest who served as their spiritual advisor. We also talked about the burgeoning pedophile scandal, and how I as a PR pro would address it, all while enjoying some of the best crab cakes in the world overlooking Baltimore's transitioning waterfront.

Ultimately, our strategic plan was adopted by the daughters, along with a slightly more humbly rendered logo—thanks to the priest's comments. My very personal peek behind the curtain came to an end; my love for and professional devotion to the daughters did not.

CHAPTER 12
OH THE HUMANITY

As much as the sisters' *human side* appealed to me, the human side of some of my coworkers and many of the ministry leaders more often repulsed me. Because we were repping for God every day, I honestly felt we owed it to all to always do our best.

I was convinced that our daily focus should be on service to our patients and their families, and that our concerns should center on the best possible medical outcomes.

The truth was that regardless of our history, tradition, and mission, we were still in the business of providing care, and health care is an *ugly* business.

Thankfully, being a mission-focused facility we attracted compassionate caregivers, leaders, and volunteers. Day in and out, caregivers at the bedside make and maintain the culture of a hospital, and most of ours did so beautifully.

Awards, accolades, and unparalleled growth and success helped convince me that we were doing *much good*. As a member of the middle management team, I was not a part of the senior leaders' regular meetings and discussions, but eventually I saw, heard, and was frequently given the task of spinning enough crazy to know there was little to no sense of *mission* at the top.

The daughters were gone, and the pack of jackals they left to run the place had run amuck.

Leaders came and went fairly quickly now, and more and more the new ones were cut from a different cloth. The kind and gentle leadership that had birthed the ministry and nurtured it for almost one hundred years was eclipsed by power-hungry type As who were in it to win it and didn't give a damn about anyone or anything else.

Extremely driven and high functioning were the primary match criteria now. Good morals, values, and ethics no longer seemed to be. Clearly, the servant-leader style, once the majority, was mostly absent among the leadership now.

Needless to say, this put me and anyone else who was still trying to be true to the daughters and their mission in great peril.

Chapter 13
Shark's Tale

On a hot Sunday afternoon in July of 2001, I received a call from a former coworker who was now working at a competitor hospital in town. She called to tell me that their facility was transferring an eight-year-old boy who had been attacked by a shark to our hospital because his condition was declining rapidly. He needed a pediatric intensive care unit. As the only children's hospital in the region, that meant he would be transferred to us.

She also told me that there was a great deal of media interest in the story, so I should be prepared. The media's interest stemmed from the unbelievable story of this boy's attack, treatment, and apparent remarkable recovery.

While fishing along the shore with his uncle, the little boy was attacked by a shark. His arm and a good part of one of his legs were torn off. Somehow, the boy's uncle managed to wrestle him free and drag him to the beach. The uncle also miraculously managed to get the shark onto the beach, where a nearby park ranger shot it, and the uncle retrieved the boy's arm.

The boy's aunt and others who had gathered on the beach as a result of all the commotion administered CPR as he lay bleeding to death while awaiting arrival of the emergency air ambulance.

The boy was flown to the hospital owned by the same company that ran the helicopter service, where he underwent more than twelve hours of surgery to reattach his severed limb and repair other life-threatening trauma he sustained.

Initially, it was reported that the boy was doing well. Official statements from the hospital to the media declared, "His reattached arm was warm and pink, and he was alert and awake."

The truth was that by Sunday, the poor little boy's kidneys were failing, and he was experiencing difficulty with a number of other internal organs due to the fact that he nearly bled to death on the beach. He was critically ill and needed serious intervention to try to stabilize his rapidly declining condition.

The national media was already well-engaged. The story was so amazing that some of the surgeons and other physicians involved in his initial care had been talking with them for nearly thirty-six hours. It was simply too spectacular for the media to walk away, and most of the physicians involved seemed more than happy to extend *their fifteen minutes*.

My first step was to meet with the boy's mother and father, who were both completely exhausted and still in shock. Worse, they felt guilty because for the first time in many years, they let someone watch their kids so they could go out for dinner to celebrate their wedding anniversary.

The whole situation was tragic. My heart hurt for all of them.

They made it clear that they wanted to avoid the media, which set the tone for the entire five weeks their son was in our care. And I, in turn, made it clear that this was the best approach, and we would *protect* them and their *privacy*.

Frankly, I was relieved that they didn't want to fuel the frenzy. Since I would be the official spokesperson with the media, we could maintain better control and present a clear and consistent message. (This became all the more important as the days wore on and more misinformation was fed to the press by some of the boy's first team of physicians.)

My first priority was the little boy—our patient—and his family, and how I was going to live up to my promise.

The truth was there was no preparing for the media circus that followed over the next five days, and nothing in my previous experience had prepared me for the world's media at our door.

National media began arriving at 5 a.m. to do live standups in front of our facility. In the first few hours of that first morning, I fielded local media calls and did live telephone interviews with radio stations in England, Australia, and Mexico. By the third day we had received over five hundred telephone calls from media and the general public.

Large gift baskets and floral arrangements from Diane Sawyer and Maury Povich were accompanied by handwritten notes asking for a personal interview. The family did not budge, and neither did we.

We had nine other children in our pediatric ICU at the time, and the same team of doctors and nurses that was caring for this little boy was also treating them. In addition, beyond the children's hospital, our facility was a full-service, regional medical center. We had hundreds of patients in our hospital each day and combined with visitors, staff, and outpatients, thousands more on the campus each day.

Our concern and need was continuing to run a smooth operation for the entire facility while managing this insatiable demand for information and footage.

Initially, we decided to provide three briefings a day to meet the media's need for fresh updates during their prime viewing times. The first two on the first day—at 7:30 a.m. and 3:00 p.m.— only consisted of me and members of the treatment team at our facility; the third, at 7:30 p.m., included members of the air ambulance and original surgical team.

The media was fixated on the boy's arm and kept asking questions about it. Our doctors tried to explain the full extent of his injuries, but that didn't fit their *sensational* story. The lead pediatric intensivist on our team explained that the arm was the least of this boy's troubles. He was experiencing more life-threatening complications of the attack, including damage to his kidneys, lungs, and brain.

The truth was the boy was critically ill and *only time would tell.*

Our entire organization seemed committed to this boy, his family, and the nine other children and their families that were also in our pediatric ICU. The truth was that while his little boy was in critical condition, he wasn't the sickest child in our hospital that day. We had babies and toddlers literally dying upstairs, and we needed to be sensitive to everyone's privacy and emotional needs.

Our challenges were made greater by the fact that a couple of the surgeons who had participated in the boy's original care were doing on-air interviews because our guys weren't.

The media seems to always find a way to tell the story *they* want.

During the first week of the boy's lengthy stay with us, one surgeon who assisted in his initial surgeries reported to the media that she had just visited the boy and "He was awake, making eye contact, and moving around." To sweeten it more so, she added, "He even smiled when shown his favorite candy bar."

None of this was true.

Nonetheless, misinformation was being spread to the media—triggering more inquiries and clarifications from us.

After the quip about the candy bar, we began to receive candy bars in the mail, along with the growing number of cards, letters, stuffed animals, gift baskets, and flowers. One letter made it with no return address and written only "To the boy who was bit by a shark in Florida" scrawled in childlike handwriting.

We had a website, which until then had been mostly underutilized, and a robust phone system, so after the first several hundred telephone inquiries, we chose to record updates that could be easily accessed by anyone and posted a written version of the same on our website. We included additional resources and information about donating to his family in order to help offset what were sure to be devastating, long-term expenses.

By the end of the first week, it was clear to all that this boy's story was not the success originally reported. At best, he was in for a long recovery. Ultimately, the media moved on.

A few more weeks passed, and the little boy improved enough to go home. Without the glare of the media spotlight, we were able to quietly arrange for home care, a combination of nursing and physical and speech therapy, and an ambulance for the trip back to his home state.

Unfortunately, someone on the receiving end of the operation leaked the news to the media, triggering another flurry of cameras and reporters as the ambulance pulled away from our facility.

I had very mixed emotions. My heart still hurt. Truthfully, I was proud of our team and all of our efforts to care for this little boy and his family; however, I was also very conflicted about sending him home.

I had successfully spun this story over several weeks to position our facility as a loving family of professionals all united in our mission and actions to provide loving, supportive care. The truth was that the entire experience made me sick to my stomach and helped me realize that at best we were a horribly dysfunctional family, with all the crazy drama that comes along with that. But my job was to preserve, protect, and further the reputation of the institution, and once again, I did so too well.

The entire situation also caused me to question modern medicine's ability to treat life-threatening traumas, terminal illness, and extremely premature births. I honestly didn't see a bright future for this poor child or his family and wondered if it wouldn't have been better if he hadn't survived the attack.

For the first time in my career, I began to question the abilities of modern care. I struggled with the fact that everything seems to be about keeping the patient alive, and no one seems to talk honestly about the *quality of life* for extremely ill patients.

It would not be the last time I visited this question.

One can't blame the clinicians. They are trained to keep people *alive*. One can't blame the loved ones of these very sick people either. Pretty much every one of us would ask a doctor to *do whatever it takes* to keep our loved ones alive.

It's simply another flaw in our current health care model.

Truthfully, there isn't enough information provided to loved ones to make *informed decisions,* and there isn't a culture in our society or medicine today that helps us to better understand when *it's time to let go.*

CHAPTER 14
MOVE ALONG, LITTLE DOGGIE

The devastation and personal loss caused by the back-to-back hurricane seasons of 2004 and 2005 coupled with the reality that I was fighting a losing battle at work felt like a sign from God that it was time to move on. I began my search to leave the health ministry that wasn't and find a better future for me and my family somewhere reasonably warm and preferably, off the coast.

I had hoped to leave the health care industry altogether, but by then my resume was fairly health care–specific. In addition, recruiting had become an automated, online function—initially involving little to no actual human contact—so I didn't seem to be able to clear the application filter systems outside of the industry.

Eventually, I had three separate opportunities for which I was being considered. One was with a venture capital start-up company that was going to be developing standalone bariatric surgery centers, another was with another large Catholic health system based in Colorado, and the third was with a small, faith-based community hospital in central Texas.

The venture capital interview was interesting, but I knew in my heart it wasn't a good fit. Similarly the interview in Denver left me with a familiar ping in my gut. The telephone call from the CEO of the little, faith-based hospital was impressive and the follow-up in person interview even more so. This guy was the real deal. Unlike many CEOs, he had the ability to actively listen.

His vision for the future looked very much like my past. The work would be easy. I would be a member of the senior management team, reporting directly to him. There would be no VP repping or directing me to carry out his/her own agenda.

We clearly connected, and I knew I could work with him. Despite my hesitancy about continuing to work in health care, *this* felt right. I happily accepted the offer and began preparations to relocate my family.

CHAPTER 15
MY GOD'S BETTER THAN YOURS

I started my new job in the dead of winter. Because my wife and youngest son stayed in Florida to sell the house before joining me, I took an apartment not far from the hospital's campus. Ironically my particular unit faced the hospital, so I literally never got away from the place for the first five months of my experience there.

It wasn't such a bad thing. I'd always been a bit of a workaholic, and with no distractions I was able to make a big impact in a very short time. I immediately set about rebranding the sleepy little community hospital both internally and externally.

I pulled out all my usual tricks and tactics. With each success my new boss was more and more pleased. He would often gush at our weekly president's council meetings. He'd send out glowing e-mails to our leadership team about the latest change or improvement—significantly crediting me for whatever it was.

Honestly, I wasn't used to praise—especially publically. It made me uncomfortable. I asked him to stop, but the guy *loved* me. I *was* making a difference, and he continued to *gush*.

Naturally, I enjoyed his validation, but I could also see what it was doing to my relationships with peers and others at the hospital. I was a bit surprised that my colleagues didn't see our wins and successes as *institutional wins* to be celebrated by all.

There were fewer than fifty folks on the leadership team, so it was easy to establish personal relationships with practically all of them. However, as I attempted to do so, with the exception of a very few, I heard *extremely* negative things about the facility, our medical staff, their coworkers, and worse, *our patients.*

It seemed clear that our mission was merely a set of words on the wall with little relevance to our day-to-day actions. I knew the impact of focusing on the health ministry aspect and highlighting our mission had on transforming the culture at my previous institution, so I set about to do the same here.

The effort worked *again.*

From staff to patients to the greater community, our facility was more and more being seen as a health ministry versus a hospital, and the benefits were significant. Many of us felt a greater sense of purpose in our daily work. Patients began remarking about the friendly attitudes of our staff, and the community took note.

Soon we were recognized as business of the year by the local Chamber of Commerce, followed by the green business of the year honors the next. The city then followed suit by bestowing a Pioneer Spirit Award on us a few years after that. We garnered best hospital honors in the local newspaper's annual people's choice awards four consecutive years in a row.

Patient volumes increased, patient satisfaction scores improved, and donations to our facility's foundation grew.

Mission outreach efforts also expanded from a single mission trip to Honduras each year and an annual employee giving campaign to hands-on, local efforts. From building wheelchair ramps for the disabled to volunteering at the local food bank to impromptu toy, clothing, food, and book drives, our mission culture was evolving, and for most of us it was a very good thing.

Shortly after overseeing a multimillion-dollar expansion and renovation, my gushing boss, the CEO, hit the wall. He felt he had done all he could and wanted to end his tenure on a high note and abruptly announced his resignation.

I knew at that moment my life would never be quite the same at this institution. I also loved where I lived and the life my wife, and now the rest of our relocated immediate family, had built in the area. I wasn't going anywhere.

Our new CEO arrived several months later. In the interim our senior leadership team and meetings had fallen apart. By the time we had our first meeting led by the new guy, we were no longer acting as a team, and it was clear we were headed in a whole new, uncharted direction.

We'd gone from a respectful, professional work environment led by an engaged, mature, and devout leader to *Lord of the Flies* meets *Animal House*. Without a leader our team had lost its way, and suddenly this thirty-something, newly minted and visibly uncomfortable "senior" leader was at the helm.

During his first year, our new CEO left things pretty much alone. He didn't start rearranging his world by eliminating any of his direct reports until twelve months had passed. The kid was smart enough to recognize his strongest players, and whether he liked us or not, he knew enough to leave us alone—initially. We, in turn, knew our day would also come.

A few years later, my day came. I left the ministry. Suffice it to say that, despite their fairly regular assertions that they were better Christians, just as I'd experienced in faith-based Catholic health care, the Adventists seem to only apply faith when convenient and mostly to defend their tax-exempt status.

Once again my words, images, ideas, and day-to-day actions helped a health system grow and prosper in spite of itself, and I felt the same guilt and shame for having contributed to the effort.

Part 4:

TAKEAWAYS

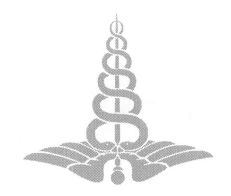

CHAPTER 16
A FOND FAREWELL

After suffering from the aftereffects of a major stroke ten years earlier, my father finally succumbed to death at eight-nine. It happened after a two-week stay in a residential hospice facility with my mom and all five siblings present.

While difficult, it was a strangely beautiful experience.

Mom had been caring for Dad at home by herself for nine years following his stroke before *finally* accepting some assistance. Appeals from me and my brothers and sister to allow occasional help for a housekeeper, meals on wheels, or even an adult daycare worker were rejected.

Dad's age and progressive loss of mobility eventually became too much for my four-foot-eleven mother to handle. A friend of my wife's who is a nurse helped us arrange for in-home nursing care and the proper equipment to make things easier for both of them via a local hospice agency.

The services were covered by insurance and a welcome change to the traditional health care grind Mom and Dad had been caught up in for nearly a decade. Hospice caregivers visited a few times a week to bathe Dad, monitor his medications—which were now fewer—and draw routine blood samples.

Though she wasn't happy about it, Mom grew to appreciate the assistance and was especially grateful that she no longer had to load Dad into the car for regular trips to the doctor and lab. The wheelchair she had fought because she feared Dad would become dependent on it made day-to-day existence easier for both of them.

Over the next year, Dad's abilities continued to decline, and he fell a few times. One particular fall happened just before his hospice aide arrived for a visit. When she saw Dad and Mom and the anxiety and stress the fall had produced, the aide immediately ordered something called respite care.

Basically this meant Dad was going to stay in residential hospice facility, and Mom and my two older brothers, who were both now providing assistance on a regular basis as well, were going to get a much-needed physical and emotional break. The respite was also covered by insurance and could last as long as two weeks.

The hospice home had been built a few years earlier specifically for inpatient care. It was small, private and beautiful appointed. It looked like a home with handsomely landscaped grounds featuring several private, lush and tranquil garden spaces for patients and/or visiting loved ones to find quiet and peace. A large, common great room included a fireplace and a never-ending supply of snacks and beverages for visitors who were also allowed to come and go 24–7.

Each private room featured high-end, home-like furnishings and artfully arranged accessories. A friendly and engaged staff of caregivers and volunteers made sure that Dad enjoyed three wonderful meals a day as well as all the snacks he wanted. They also visited regularly to see if he needed anything more and checked on Mom and my brothers as well.

It wasn't traditional health care. It was loving *comfort* care.

Veteran's Day happened to fall shortly after Dad arrived at the home. He was treated to even more special attention as a WWII vet. Dad was pleased. He knew the stay was temporary, and he'd always been a sucker for lots of care and attention. By the end of his first week, though, his health started to decline rapidly. He was beginning to experience organ failure.

My sister had already flown down to assist. My younger brother and I checked in with my mom by phone daily, and as she had throughout the past ten years, she downplayed the full extent of Dad's situation. By then he was in and out of conscious.

Thankfully, my oldest brother called to tell me what was really going on, and I left early the next morning for the eleven-hour trek back to Florida. I was grateful to arrive in time to spend a few minutes alone with Dad the morning after I arrived. He was awake and aware. We hugged, chatted briefly, and told each other, "I love you." Then he fell asleep—never to fully awake again.

My younger brother arrived the next day, and for the reminder of it and most of the next, all five siblings gathered together along with Mom in Dad's room. We took turns rubbing his shoulders, patting his chest, hands and feet, and letting him know his loving family was there with him. The soundtrack of Dad's life played quietly in the background via a set of songs he had my wife prepare a year or so earlier to be played during his memorial service. Thankfully, he had previously directed us to make it an upbeat celebration of his life rather than a traditional funeral.

It was the first time only the seven of us had been alone together in more than forty years. It was quiet, peaceful, and loving. By the end of the second night of our vigil, with all of us gathered around him, Dad gently passed.

With the exception of an IV, there was little evidence of medical intervention. Staff was present but kept a quiet, respectful distance. No one came in hourly and turned on bright lights to take vitals or lab samples. There was no steady stream of people coming and going from his room. And no one came by each day to visit and ask about our patient experience.

The time we spent there was about us and our needs, not the institution's heavy-handed attempts to improve its scores and in turn, its reimbursement rates.

I was grateful for the time we had together and the beautiful way the hospice home and its staff attended to the needs of all of us before, during, and after Dad's death. I thought about how lucky we all were to have experienced death in such a peaceful, loving way. And I wondered again why more doctors, caregivers, and loved ones don't look into hospice *sooner.*

Dad began receiving in-home hospice long before he was dying. The comfort, help, and support he and Mom received during his final year made the quality of life better for *all* of us.

There's no doubt in my mind many more Americans would choose it if the American health system and society fully embraced and truly advocated for it. Rather than using it as a last resort in the final days of a "terminal situation," hospice and palliative care need to be discussed and included in treatment and care options from the beginning of the process in order for more of us to make thoughtful, informed choices.

I was grateful that Dad and I had discussed the subject of his death more than once through the years. He made it clear that he didn't want to be "kept alive" in some hospital room or nursing home with lots of machinery, tubes, and other technology, prolonging the inevitable. Both he and Mom had advanced directives on file with their health care providers as well. Sadly, many Americans fail to have these conversations with their loved ones, and none of us wants to be the one who pulls the plug on those we love.

Making your wishes known while you are healthy and aware is the best approach, and putting it into writing with your family and providers will help ensure that they are carried out as *you* directed.

Advanced directives and medical power of attorney forms are available online and through your doctor, hospital, and other care centers. You will be asked if you have them among the myriad questions with which you are bombarded prior to any medical procedure; however, you may not realize what they are or their significance.

Do yourself, your loved ones, and your providers a favor; fill them out and get them into your medical record.

CHAPTER 17
WE DON'T SPEAK YOUR LANGUAGE

Like everything else in health care today, the *language* of health care is complex. Acronyms reign supreme, and misused terms mislead and often confuse patients. Ironically, very often it's a simple communication breakdown that leads to bad outcomes in health care.

One very real example of confusing terminology comes in the form of industry job titles. While customers (patients) are meant to and often do find comfort in the following job titles, the truth is they shouldn't. During a hospitalization, your patient advocate is not really *advocating for you*, the patient. He or she is primarily employed to resolve any customer-service issues during your stay so you'll give the hospital a good rating on its patient satisfaction survey should you receive one. This is very important to the hospital because reimbursement rates today are partially based on patient satisfaction scores.

Similarly, your case manager isn't managing your case to benefit you. He or she is managing your care on behalf of the hospital to ensure maximum payment from your insurer and timely discharge to mitigate any unnecessary expenditure that will *not* be reimbursed.

Code speak and shorthand dialogue between providers in your presence only further challenges even the most intelligent among us. Terminology and concepts we use in everyday life have a different meaning in health care. For example, a negative test result in health care vernacular is generally a good thing, whereas a positive result could mean trouble.

From hospital signage to job titles to medical subspecialties, the language of health care is not at all user-friendly. While that is not uncommon—many industries have a language of their own—the difference is in health care, the code speak expands beyond provider to provider and regularly spills into direct communication with patients. And the critical difference between health care and other industries is that miscommunications cost people their health and in some cases, their lives.

There is a sound logic to the language of health care. It works and is necessary between caregivers; however, there needs to be more than one language spoken in health care, and the industry is very slow to recognize this and adapt accordingly.

The best health outcomes are achieved when patient and provider have good, effective, two-way communication. This ideal is difficult to achieve for a variety of reasons, but the industry simply must work harder to ensure that it happens for *every* patient during *every* encounter.

The additional barriers between a non-English-speaking patient and his or her health provider(s) further complicates the vital, two-way communication needed between patient and provider. Very often the English-speaking children of a patient are used to communicate with their loved ones. While this seems like a viable solution, the truth is it is not.

The disabled, the chronically infirm, the elderly, and the very young are among health care's biggest clientele, and yet, to date, health care is failing to ensure that every patient—regardless of origin and social, economic, or health status—is ensured *effective, two-way communication.*

When a loved one can't interpret, hospitals turn to other staff—housekeepers, office workers, etc.—to translate. They have the option of employing translator services, including online models, but to contain costs, they generally don't turn on the service unless the patient specifically asks for it. Like so many other situations in health care, most patients don't know they have a right to do so.

Would you want a receptionist, housekeeper, cafeteria worker, or insurance clerk short-handing vital communication that could save your life?

We all played the telephone game as kids. We'd laugh about how mixed up the communication got when translated and rephrased from person to person. Now imagine having to explain a complicated medical procedure, treatment options, lifestyle changes, etc., to a loved one.

There is nothing funny about miscommunication in health care.

This very real problem is occurring all day, every day in doctors' offices and hospitals across America. Until the health care industry commits to effective, two-way communication for all, potential misdiagnosis and ultimate mistreatment will continue to cost Americans their good health and some cases, their lives.

In the insurance world, intentionally misleading terms and labels further confuse the unsuspecting public. Insurance reforms brought about by the Affordable Care Act make it even harder to unscramble the alphabet soup of health plan options.

Misleading terms like health maintenance organization (HMO), preferred provider organization (PPO), as well as exclusive provider organization (EPO), to name but a few, suggest that these types of plans are focused on maintaining your health or providing preferred, exclusive, or better care when in fact that's not the focus of the plans or these engineered groups at all.

When you break it all down, all these models are fairly similar in that they are *not about you*. Each model uses a predetermined group of providers who have negotiated with the insurer to accept a certain rate and agree to provide care to you within the guidelines of the particular plan.

Despite the misleading product names and movie-quality TV ads, *all* insurance plans are designed to keep costs down by denying and/or limiting the care you receive.

If you are shopping for a new insurance plan—for whatever reason—do the research! Understand how the plan you are looking at actually works, what's covered and what's not, which doctors and other providers are in the plan, and which hospital(s) and emergency rooms you may use under the plan.

You also need to look closely at your annual out-of-pocket expenses. Plans that appear more affordable due to a low monthly premium often end up costing the user more because of high deductibles and copays per encounter.

Last, your health status should help you determine which plan to purchase. For example, if you're a diabetic on insulin daily, your plan needs to cover diabetes treatment and prescriptions.

I know this seems obvious, but you'll thank me later.

We can and must do better. Health care consumers have to become better informed, active participants in their health and demand that their rights to effective communication be met.

CHAPTER 18
DANCING WITH THE DEVIL

To be clear, I do not believe doctors are inherently bad people who set out to do you harm. I do believe the current/ traditional health care delivery model gives entirely too much power and control to doctors. It's not entirely their fault. Most Americans happily turn themselves completely over to their doctors to be fixed, and many doctors take full advantage of this *misplaced trust.*

I have worked with some wonderful doctors through the years. The ones that stand out to me are not only good medical practitioners but also good communicators. The good ones focus on showing you how much they care rather than how much they know. You know, the fully rounded, human ones.

Shortly before leaving my last hospital job, I ran into the president of our medical staff while rounding on patients. He was one of the good guys. Great clinician, smart, focused, compassionate. He stopped me to inquire about my wife's health. He had performed some of her diagnostic testing a year before to rule out any cardiac issues. I was pleased and not surprised that he cared enough to ask, thanked him for his inquiry and shared that things really weren't any better. I also shared that I felt the care and some of the prescriptions were making her situation worse, so we were moving away from the specialists and heavy duty drugs toward lifestyle changes and alternative therapies.

Without skipping a beat, he said, "That's smart. Keep her away from doctors and hospitals."

Unfortunately, just like all other walks of life, fully rounded, healthy beings are few and far between. All of life's dysfunctions run rampant in health care, but the byproduct is far more dangerous.

Honestly, I've known practitioners who were almost like idiot savants—brilliant in one area of their lives and hopelessly lacking in all others. I think this is another major flaw in modern health care. The truth is that certain personality traits along with a right-brained focus are what make for a great clinician. The challenge is these alone are not the skills required for the compassionate partner you want and need to accompany you on your health care journey.

All the more reason we, the *patients* need to become *consumers* of health care services. We must shop, research, become our own experts on and price/quality, and compare our health care choices and spending, just like everything else of any significance on which we spend our money.

Sadly, most of us spend more time researching our smartphone purchases than we do on our health purchases. And ironically, very few of us make use of the numerous, free, and helpful health apps now available through our phones.

So you've seen behind the curtain. *Doctors aren't who you thought they were.*

Unfortunately you can't avoid them—entirely. Eventually, we all have to dance with these "devils." If you must seek care, be smart about it. Here are a number of helpful tips compiled from a variety of sources through my years of producing patient literature and magazine articles that really resonate.

If you have some sort of chronic condition that already requires regular visits with a physician and ongoing prescriptions, you'll want a primary care physician. Choosing the right one requires you to look beyond his/her medical credentials—although you do need to check those out. Thankfully today there are several free national websites that allow you to research a doctor. Safety records, outcomes, and even patient experience data are all available for your review at no cost online.

Once you've found a doctor who passes the credentials test, there are a few other key points to consider.

- Compatibility: Do you and your doctor have similar interests, likes, and hobbies? Do you feel a connection with him/her?
- Accessibility: How conveniently located is his/her office to your home/workplace? What about the practice's hours? Is it open when you're likely to need use it?
- Specialty/Hospital Support: Is he/she part of a larger group? Does the group contain medical subspecialists? To which hospital does he/she admit?
- Expertise: Regardless of why you are seeing a physician, you need to know his/her true expertise. Many doctors today offer a variety of services—some beyond their board certification. When you need care, be sure to investigate that particular provider's experience. You can find information about any provider, including his or her outcomes, online. And just like the auto mechanic, you want the physician who does whatever it is you need to be doing it frequently and well.

By the way, all of these same criteria should be applied to any hospital, care facility, and/or outpatient treatment center at which you are considering receiving care. Online ratings are also available. (Don't just go to the perspective facility's website; go to an impartial, qualified reviewer to get the whole truth.)

Your best health outcomes will be the result of your personal efforts *in collaboration* with your doctor. Proven research shows that good doctor-patient relations result in happier and healthier patients. From decreased blood pressure to reduced stress to building trusting, two-way relationships, studies show that improved outcomes are the result of good communication with one's doctor.

Good communication with your doctor is not easy. You must overcome your intimidation of their world, language, and implied authority. When you're going see a doctor, make a list of symptoms and questions before your visit.

First, remember that your communication needs to be respectful, friendly, and open if you expect the same in return. During the appointment, do the following:

- Ask questions.
- If you are unclear about something your doctor or his/her nurse said, ask him/her to explain it. Have him/her break it down in layman's terms.
- Take notes during your visit.
- Ideally, if you can bring a close friend or loved one with you, that's even better. A second set of ears—especially one that isn't compromised by whatever brought you to the doctor's office—is extremely helpful.
- When you get home, review your notes, and do some online research on what you were told.
- Check into side effects and contraindications of any prescriptions, and be prepared to talk with your doctor about any of it that concerns you. *Do not* wait until your follow-up appointment. Call your doctor's office and express your concerns. If you do not feel comfortable with what you heard or read, do not proceed with that course of treatment without first speaking to your doctor.

Ultimately, maintaining good health is your best offense against unnecessary encounters with doctors. To minimize your exposure to doctors, practice good preventive health habits, lead a healthy lifestyle, know your health risk factors, and know your important numbers, like blood pressure, sugar, cholesterol, and weight. But mostly, don't be too humble or intimidated when dealing with a doctor.

It's your health and your life, and it's honestly *just a job* to your doctor and the rest of the caregivers you see.

CHAPTER 19
HEALTHY U

"**Y**ou're so lucky."
"You don't look (insert whatever age I am at the time)!"
"Do you eat *like that all* the time?"

For most of my life, people have made comments about my appearance. The truth is I almost always felt I had nothing to do with it. From the way I look to my skills and my good health genes, I always viewed myself as an inheritance from my parents. There's longevity and relatively good health on both sides of my family. But as I've gotten older, I realize I made lots of choices along the way that have contributed to my "luck" and good health.

Initially, it wasn't so much *my* choice. Both my parents were very concerned with image as we were growing up. For my dad in particular, image was everything. Growing up in the Depression contributed to this belief; being a part of the *Mad Men* world as an advertising executive in the '60s and '70s only reaffirmed the concept for him.

Like many postwar, middle class American males, my father's lovely home, new car every few years, and fashionable wardrobe were measures of his success. A beautiful wife and a handsome brood raised the stakes with his competitors a bit more.

Both my parents made lots of remarks about our looks, hair, clothing, weight, etc., on a regular basis. I learned early what was expected.

In junior high and the first half of high school, I was a competitive gymnast. Our coaches were also extremely focused on our weight, appearance, and overall fitness. By the time I was to move into the varsity squad, our team was practicing 364 days a year, and that's when I'd had enough of organized sports. No regrets. I learned about teamwork and healthy competiveness. I gained confidence, self-discipline, and a lifetime understanding of how to be physically active.

You might say genetics play into my taste preferences. As an American of mostly Italian descent, I seem to naturally prefer a lighter, more Mediterranean-style diet with lots of vegetables. And I like fish and poultry over red meat. I love salad, and when I eat sweets, I prefer them to be more savory than sugary.

Mental wellness is another area of importance, and I've been fortunate here as well. Even though most of my family, myself included, occasionally suffers from some sort of depression, I've received a great deal of training and education focused on leadership and being the best you can be through the years. The Catholic health system focused on learning more about ourselves. From servant leadership and the Keirsey Temperament Sorter to Myers Briggs, John Maxwell, and Quint Studer, I spent many hours thinking about whom I was and what motivates or demotivates me. I learned that genetics play a role in who I was born as, but conscious choices I make daily shape and reshape who I am.

Too many people use genetics as their excuse for their health. You often hear things like "Both my mom and dad were big ... Diabetes, heart disease, etc., runs in my family ... I grew up in *(insert region)*. I don't eat that."

There's an expression in health care that makes the tired excuse of poor health being your *birthright* no longer valid. The saying goes, "Genetics loads the gun; lifestyle pulls the trigger." In other words, while you may be predisposed to be overweight, diabetic, addicted to something, etc., your day-to-day actions and behaviors can overcome that prescribed version of your life.

During my last stint with a hospital, I learned a great deal about their particular faith's health habits, which date back to the formation of the faith. Their healthy lifestyle is credited with helping many of them live to a healthy and more vibrant old age. *National Geographic* did a cover story on it. A book titled *The Blue Zones* explored the phenomenon, and Oprah Winfrey did a TV special on it as well. Documented evidence shows that certain cultures around the world, including some in America, choose to lead a certain type of lifestyle, and it contributes to a longer and healthier life.

Our hospital parent began teaching and promoting their healthy living philosophies via a lifestyle program they developed a few years after I joined the team. The program featured an acronym that spelled out eight major principles that make up the lifestyle.

I was tapped to become our local ministry's healthy living leader and attended workshops and eventually taught the philosophies to others. I liked and identified with the program and its philosophies because of the simplicity of the concepts and the ease with which one can learn to live it.

I taught healthy living concepts to coworkers and community members via workshops, and because I was talking the talk, I made a point to walk the walk. The eight principles worked for me and many others to whom I helped teach them. Stories of healthy and permanent weight loss, improved sleep patterns, and the resulting improved outlook on life, and for some getting off all of their prescription medications, were often shared.

The truth is there are many good models and cultures from whom we can learn to live in a much healthier fashion, but for the most part everything I've read, researched, written, taught, and tried to practice suggests that healthy living all boils down to a balanced lifestyle that features eating right, staying reasonably physically and mentally active, remaining positive and hopeful, enjoying hobbies, interests, and other people, and getting the right amount and type of rest.

As easy as that sounds, it's not easy to accomplish.

The challenge with healthy living is the concept isn't embraced by the medical community or for that matter, American culture at large. Today, if one chooses to live and eat healthy, one is forced to live an *alternative* lifestyle. Since we changed eating habits because of my wife's illness, I've become acutely aware of the food industry's failure to help us eat better and properly. Misleading labeling, deceptive marketing practices, and feeding into the American culture of "more is better" all contribute to the challenge.

Modern medicine isn't helping either. Medical practitioners and health care institutions all make money *treating sick people.* There is no money in wellness for today's medical industrial complex.

In addition, all of the other industries that benefit from your poor health and/or belief that you need them and their products in order to achieve good health aren't truly focused on you either. They are all *selling* you something to improve your health, looks, and attitude, and shame on you, you're buying it.

Long-term good health doesn't come in a box. It doesn't require a special outfit, major equipment, or a membership to anything. Good health doesn't come from a surgical enhancement or the latest miracle pill, drink, or gadget that Dr. Oz and countless others hawk daily.

Sustainable good health comes from you; only you can make it happen. Better health begins with you being completely honest with yourself. You need to be realistic about what you like and don't, what you're willing to do and not. You need to consider your whole life—work, family, social and recreational activities, your relationships, eating and other habits, etc. Then you need to make small, meaningful changes to begin a healthier path. It's about developing a realistic lifestyle that you can and *will* follow. And when you don't, you need to forgive yourself and try again.

Eventually your improved mood, looks, and physical abilities, along with the compliments you will receive from others for them, will sustain you and keep you focused on staying on the path.

Be nice. Don't be overly hard on yourself or others (who made you screw up). And give it time. You didn't get in poor health overnight, and you won't be living healthy immediately either. Long-term success requires discipline, patience, humor, balance, and lots of forgiveness of yourself and others.

Resources on the subject are limitless. Do your own research. Don't believe the marketing and advertising hype of anything. Read labels. Consult reputable, nonbiased, and ideally unpaid sources. Become educated on wellness, and then develop the plan and path you can follow for the rest of your healthy existence.

CHAPTER 20
THE TIME IS NOW

O ver a thirty-year span I contributed to furthering the myth that the American health care system works and works well. I helped to shape perceptions and drive business into the intuitions for which I worked. I kidded myself into believing that the truths I shared were the *only* truths. I chose to focus on the positive aspects of the growth in mission outreach and good works and the development of new and needed services. I justified what I did each day by knowing I did my best to make the things I promoted and shared *true*. And the truth is they were, but they weren't the *only* truths.

I only had so much air time and attention span with the audiences I was charged with influencing, so like any good PR pro, I made the most of the stories and opportunities that portrayed our compassion and positive outcomes and sold our best and most profitable services.

The *whole* truth is that today's antiquated, bloated, and ineffective American health system is ill-prepared and ill-equipped to take on Obamacare or the Ebola crisis or any other wide-scale challenge. The politics, economics, and responsibilities of the American health care system today are in major crisis.

While the concept of universal health care and a single-payer system may sound appealing, I can say with absolute certainty and total honesty that the current processes, protocols, and attitudes of the health care industry simply cannot deliver on the promise.

The 2016 election cycle is already in full swing and health care reform has only briefly been mentioned so far. It's important that we change the focus and debate from the two parties' talking points to a full-fledged investigation of the health care industry's successes and failures.

The discussion must be all encompassing, constructive, and relentless in its efforts to truly fix the major gaps, shortcomings, and critical failures of the current model.

True, comprehensive change and improvement cannot be squeezed into an election cycle or single legislative term. The current health care model is institutionalized medicine, and like the outdated education and banking systems in America, it's based on old and very tired models.

The reforms brought about by the Affordable Care Act are a beginning, but providing *more access* to a broken, ineffective, and outdated model of care isn't the proper solution.

Worse, there's very little affordable about the coverage available as a result of the act. Research I recently conducted for a plan comparable to the one provided my employer was going to run close to $700 per month in premiums and require that we meet a $12,000 annual deductible *before* any coverage kicked in.

Reforms focusing on insurance companies such as preexisting conditions, preventive services, and dependent coverage were all good outcomes, but much more needs to be done to rein in the control and profits of these corporate killers.

In addition, today's medical industrial complex is much too focused on only treating *sick people*. Little to no attention is paid to wellness and prevention. Lifestyle and nutrition are very recent additions to the health care mind-set, and many older practitioners—those who have been out of school for ten or more years—*still* give it no credence. Similarly, despite growing evidence outside of the mainstream medical establishment, absolutely no credence or recognition is given to supplements and so-called alternative therapies either.

Reform must be developed from the perspective of the greater good of all. The ugly truth is the current model isn't working—for Democrats and Republicans alike, those with insurance and those without.

Truthfully, most doctors, nurses, and other caregivers—even individual hospitals—will tell you the current state of care isn't working for them either. The only ones seeming to be benefiting from today's health care model are insurance and pharmaceutical companies, health care corporations, manufacturers of medical equipment and supplies, and each of their respective lobbyists.

Health care in America isn't working, because very few in the industry are actually and *honestly* working to make it work for you, the consumer/patient. *Why would those in control of health care in America work to change it when it's working for them?*

In addition, because alternative therapies and innovative care delivery models aren't recognized by and, in turn, are not paid for by insurance, there's little incentive for traditional medicine to explore and adopt these and other proven practices, or delivery models.

Despite this disincentive, more and more Americans, like my wife and I, have found better health avoiding traditional models and mindsets. We now look to alternative medicines and practices *first*.

All health care systems today are designed to meet national safety and quality standards (in order to receive payment for services rendered), as well as the budgetary and other corporate measures instilled by the particular facility's owner. In other words, it truly is *all about the bottom line.*

Seldom are system changes and governmental regulations designed to actually meet the needs of the consumer/patient.

Worse, in spite of twenty-first-century advances, by and large, health care is still following protocols and practices that were put in place in the midtwentieth century or *earlier.*

Inefficiencies, bad outcomes, and major inequalities in focus of services continue to illustrate the medical industrial complex's failure to meet its commitments to the various populations and communities it serves.

The time to act is *now*.

The government is not going to solve this problem unless *we*, the American public, force it to. Change will only occur when we begin to change the way *we* view, utilize, access, define, and pay for health care services.

Imagine what could happen if the public stopped accepting and supporting the system as it is. As the old saying goes, information is power, and too many Americans today are willing to accept advertising as fact, misinformation as truth, and an unrealistic, photo-shopped, and idealized version of health, youthfulness, and beauty as *real*.

From health-and-wellness education to the food industry to the media, government, and ultimately, industrialized health care itself, change is possible. It's also necessary and could prove to be a huge factor in improving not only our personal and collective health and well-being but also our national economy.

Once unshackled by its current mind-set, a new truthful, broader, and healthier ideal of what good health, proper nutrition, and necessary lifestyles are would no doubt create innovation, opportunities, product and service development, and new jobs and peripheral industries for many more.

The best prescription for what truly ails America could be an honest, redirected focus on health and well-being.

Ironically, my generation—the Baby Boomers—has begun regularly accessing health care and, if they haven't already, will soon learn the system doesn't work the way they thought. It's time for the same energy and spirit that helped end the Vietnam War and usher in the sexual revolution and the women's movement to rise up once again and demand a new, better way for all.

The Millennials should be equally concerned about yet another American institution that has already, and will continue to fail them.

Wake up. Act out. It's time for a revolution.

The power and speed with which change can occur in our country, thanks to the free exchange of ideas and information via the internet, make a true health care revolution *possible*. Handheld health care is here and needs to be utilized to its full potential. The development of additional alternative delivery models and methods could spark America's greatest century of ingenuity and economic development. Handled correctly, the outcome could be even more significant to the long-term viability of this country than the original American Revolution. After all, freedom without one's health is anything but free.

Sadly, today's health care model that we Boomers are now beginning to use is *still* our mama's health care, and she, and we, all deserve better.

Printed in the United States
By Bookmasters